the

Healing

Protocol

Journal

A journal for tracking your progress through an elimination diet, including GAPS, AIP, low FODMAPS and more

MICHELLE BROWN, CTNC

This work is for informational purposes only and is not intended to be a substitute for professional medical advice. It is advised to consult a medical professional before making any changes to your diet. Use the information in this book at your own risk.

Welcome!

m so excited that you've grabbed the Healing Protocol Journal, and I hope you are too! Although, let's face it, starting a strict elimination diet isn't what most people would call "exciting." Who wants to restrict their diet and give up some of their favorite foods?

An elimination diet can be tough, but I'm here to tell you that if you're currently struggling with some serious health issues- autoimmune disease, depression, anxiety, hormone imbalance, digestive problems like IBS, or what have you- a healing protocol that eliminates inflammatory foods can make a world of difference!

It certainly has for me. Diagnosed with Hashimoto's Thyroiditis in my early 20's, I wasn't given any real answers to my thyroid dysfunction, joint pain, brain fog, exhaustion and depression- until I discovered the Paleo diet.

When I cut gluten, dairy products and soy from my diet I was amazed at what happened next. My joint pain, mouth sores and digestive issues cleared up. I started to feel more clear headed and energetic.

But truth be told, I still had some work to do. My digestive tract wasn't healthy. I had a gut infection that was causing leaky gut and triggering autoimmunity. I learned that I had to really dial in my nutrition to eliminate other inflammatory foods that were continuing to irritate my system.

I also found that I needed to learn to relax, reduce my stress level, prioritize sleep and get plenty of exercise, fresh air, and sunshine. It took some work, but I can attest that every change was totally worth it.

So, yes, my friend, it's time to get excited! You've got a full life of beautiful memories to make that are going to require plenty of energy, clear thinking, and vibrant health. This healing journey just may the best thing you'll ever do, too. Let's get started!

Michelle

overcomingauto.com

How To Use This Journal

WEEKLY PROGRESS TRACKER
I've found that it can be really powerful to be able to track your progress on a weekly basis, as well as daily. It's helpful to be able to look back over the course of a few weeks or months at a glance and see how far you've come. Use this section to track your progress and setbacks so you can stay motivated.

REINTRODUCTION TRACKER
Remember, elimination diets aren't meant to last forever! As your body heals you'll be adding foods back into your diet and watching for symptoms of food sensitivities. Keep track of which foods you're introducing and your reactions all in one handy place.

DAILY FOOD & MOOD JOURNAL
Here's where you will track your daily meals, your mood, physical symptoms and bowel movements as well as sleep, or any other issues you wish to track. Keeping track of the foods I ate and how they were affecting me made a huge difference in my progress through an elimination diet. You will be able to quickly identify food sensitivities and problem foods if you really take the time to pay attention to the way your body reacts to the foods your are consuming.

I purposely left plenty of room for you to write and to adapt the journal to your own style. This is YOUR tool to track your progress on your healing journey. I encourage you to make it personal and use it in a way that fits you best!

NEED MORE HELP GETTING STARTED?
I've created a short video to show you how to use The Healing Protocol Journal. You can find it at: www.overcomingauto.com/healingprotocol. You will also find a 15 page guide to navigating elimination diets, including Guidelines for each healing protocol, a Supplements Checklist, a Healing Basics Checklist and much more! Hop over there and grab these free resources as my gift to you.

Notes

Weekly Progress Tracker

Week of: Progress/ Setbacks

_____
_____
_____
_____
❀
_____
_____
_____
_____
❀
_____
_____
_____
_____
❀
_____
_____
_____
_____
❀
_____
_____
_____
_____
❀
_____
_____
_____
_____

Weekly Progress Tracker

Week of: Progress/ Setbacks

_____
_____
_____
❖
_____
_____
_____
❖
_____
_____
_____
❖
_____
_____
_____
❖
_____
_____
_____
❖
_____
_____
_____

Re-Introduction Tracker

Food Introduced

Reactions/ Symptoms

Re-Introduction Tracker

Food Introduced

Reactions/Symptoms

Date

Meals   Mood/ Physical Symptoms

Re-Introductions:_____

Digestion

BMs: _____

Sleep/ Other Notes

Date

Meals   Mood/ Physical Symptoms

Re-Introductions:_____

Digestion

BMs: _____

Sleep/ Other Notes

Date

Meals   Mood/Physical Symptoms

❀

❀

❀

❀

Re-Introductions:_____

Digestion

BMs: _____

Sleep/Other Notes

_____

_____

Date

Meals   Mood/ Physical Symptoms

_____
_____
_____
_____
_____
_____
_____
_____
_____
_____
_____
_____
_____
_____
_____
_____
_____

Re-Introductions:_____

Digestion

BMs: _____

Sleep/ Other Notes

_____
_____

Date

Meals

Mood/Physical Symptoms

❀

❀

❀

❀

Re-Introductions:_____

Digestion

BMs: _____

Sleep/ Other Notes

_____

_____

Date

Meals

Mood/ Physical Symptoms

❀

❀

❀

❀

Re-Introductions:_____

Digestion

BMs: _____

Sleep/ Other Notes

_____

_____

Date

Meals   Mood/Physical Symptoms

Re-Introductions:_____

Digestion

BMs: _____

Sleep/Other Notes

Date

Meals   Mood/ Physical Symptoms

_____
_____
_____
_____
_____
_____
_____
_____
_____
_____
_____
_____
_____
_____
_____
_____

Re-Introductions:_____

Digestion

BMs: _____

Sleep/ Other Notes

_____
_____

Date

Meals   ## Mood/ Physical Symptoms

❀

❀

❀

❀

Re-Introductions:_____

Digestion

BMs: _____

Sleep/ Other Notes

Date

Meals   Mood/ Physical Symptoms

Re-Introductions: _____

Digestion

BMs: _____

Sleep/ Other Notes

Date

Meals   ## Mood/Physical Symptoms

_____
❀
_____
_____
_____
_____
❀
_____
_____
_____
_____
❀
_____
_____
_____
_____
❀
_____
_____
_____
_____

Re-Introductions:_____

Digestion

BMs: _____

Sleep/Other Notes

_____
_____

Date

Meals   Mood/Physical Symptoms

Re-Introductions:_____

Digestion

BMs: _____

Sleep/Other Notes

Date

Meals   Mood/Physical Symptoms

✦

✦

✦

✦

Re-Introductions:_____

Digestion

BMs: _____

Sleep/Other Notes

_____

_____

Date

Meals

Mood/ Physical Symptoms

❀

❀

❀

❀

Re-Introductions:_____

Digestion

BMs: _____

Sleep/ Other Notes

_____

_____

Date

Meals

Mood/ Physical Symptoms

Re-Introductions:_____

Digestion

BMs: _____

Sleep/ Other Notes

Date

Meals   Mood/ Physical Symptoms

Re-Introductions:_____

Digestion

BMs: _____

Sleep/ Other Notes

Meals

Mood/ Physical Symptoms

_____
_____
_____
_____
_____
_____
_____
_____
_____
_____
_____
_____
_____
_____
_____
_____

Re-Introductions:_____

Digestion

BMs: _____

Sleep/ Other Notes

_____
_____

Date

Meals   Mood/ Physical Symptoms

_____
_____
_____
_____
_____
_____
_____
_____
_____
_____
_____
_____
_____
_____
_____
_____

Re-Introductions:_____

Digestion

BMs: _____

Sleep/ Other Notes

_____
_____

Date

Meals   ## Mood/ Physical Symptoms

Re-Introductions:_____

Digestion

BMs: _____

Sleep/ Other Notes

Date

Meals   ## Mood/ Physical Symptoms

_____
_____
_____
_____
_____
_____
_____
_____
_____
_____
_____
_____
_____
_____
_____
_____
_____
_____

Re-Introductions:_____

Digestion

BMs: _____

Sleep/ Other Notes

_____
_____

Date

Meals   Mood/ Physical Symptoms

❁

❁

❁

❁

Re-Introductions:_____

Digestion

BMs: _____

Sleep/ Other Notes

_____

_____

Date

Meals   Mood/ Physical Symptoms

_____
_____
_____
_____
_____
_____
_____
_____
_____
_____
_____
_____
_____
_____
_____
_____

Re-Introductions:_____

Digestion

BMs: _____

Sleep/ Other Notes

_____
_____

Meals   Mood/ Physical Symptoms

_____ _____
❁
_____ _____

_____ _____

_____ _____
❁
_____ _____

_____ _____

_____ _____
❁
_____ _____

_____ _____

_____ _____
❁
_____ _____

_____ _____

Re-Introductions:_____

Digestion

BMs: _____

Sleep/ Other Notes

_____

_____

Date

Meals

Mood/ Physical Symptoms

_____

_____

_____

_____

_____

_____

_____

_____

_____

_____

_____

_____

_____

_____

_____

Re-Introductions:_____

Digestion

BMs: _____

Sleep/ Other Notes

_____

_____

Date

Meals   Mood/ Physical Symptoms

_____
❁ _____
_____
_____
_____
_____
❁ _____
_____
_____
_____
_____
❁ _____
_____
_____
_____
_____
❁ _____
_____
_____

Re-Introductions:_____

Digestion

BMs: _____

Sleep/ Other Notes

_____
_____

Date

Meals

Mood/ Physical Symptoms

Re-Introductions:_____

Digestion

BMs: _____

Sleep/ Other Notes

Date

Meals   Mood/ Physical Symptoms

❁

❁

❁

❁

Re-Introductions:_____

Digestion

BMs: _____

Sleep/ Other Notes

Date

Meals   *Mood/Physical Symptoms*

❁

❁

❁

❁

Re-Introductions:_____

Digestion

BMs: _____

Sleep/Other Notes

Date

Meals

Mood/ Physical Symptoms

❈

❈

❈

❈

Re-Introductions:_____

Digestion

BMs: _____

Sleep/ Other Notes

Meals   *Mood/ Physical Symptoms*

_____
_____
_____
_____
_____
_____
_____
_____
_____
_____
_____
_____
_____
_____
_____
_____

Re-Introductions:_____

Digestion

BMs: _____

Sleep/ Other Notes

_____
_____

Date

Meals   Mood/ Physical Symptoms

Re-Introductions:

Digestion

BMs: _____

Sleep/ Other Notes

Date

Meals   ## Mood/ Physical Symptoms

_____
_____
_____
_____
_____
_____
_____
_____
_____
_____
_____
_____
_____
_____
_____

Re-Introductions:_____

Digestion

BMs: _____

Sleep/ Other Notes

_____
_____

Date

Meals   Mood/Physical Symptoms

Re-Introductions:_____

Digestion

BMs: _____

Sleep/Other Notes

_____

_____

Date

Meals   Mood/Physical Symptoms

Re-Introductions:_____

Digestion

BMs: _____

Sleep/Other Notes

_____

_____

Date

Meals   Mood/Physical Symptoms

❀

❀

❀

❀

Re-Introductions:_____

Digestion

BMs: _____

Sleep/Other Notes

_____

_____

Date

Meals   Mood/Physical Symptoms

_____   ❁
_____
_____
_____
_____
_____
_____   ❁
_____
_____
_____
_____
_____
_____   ❁
_____
_____
_____
_____
_____
_____   ❁
_____
_____
_____
_____

Re-Introductions:_____

Digestion

BMs: _____

Sleep/Other Notes

_____
_____

Date

Meals   Mood/Physical Symptoms

Re-Introductions:_____

Digestion

BMs: _____

Sleep/Other Notes

_____

_____

Date

Meals

Mood/Physical Symptoms

Re-Introductions: _____

Digestion

BMs: _____

Sleep/Other Notes

Date

Meals   Mood/Physical Symptoms

Re-Introductions:_____

Digestion

BMs: _____

Sleep/Other Notes

Date

Meals   ## Mood/Physical Symptoms

Re-Introductions:_____

Digestion

BMs: _____

Sleep/Other Notes

Date

Meals   Mood/ Physical Symptoms

_____
❀_____
_____
_____
_____
_____
❀_____
_____
_____
_____
_____
❀_____
_____
_____
_____
_____
❀_____
_____
_____
_____

Re-Introductions:_____

Digestion

BMs: _____

Sleep/ Other Notes

_____
_____

Date

Meals   Mood/Physical Symptoms

Re-Introductions:_____

Digestion

BMs: _____

Sleep/Other Notes

Date

Meals   Mood/ Physical Symptoms

❀

❀

❀

❀

Re-Introductions:_____

Digestion

BMs: _____

Sleep/ Other Notes

_____

_____

Date

Meals   Mood/Physical Symptoms

Re-Introductions:_____

Digestion

BMs: _____

Sleep/Other Notes

Date

Meals

Mood/Physical Symptoms

Re-Introductions:_____

Digestion

BMs: _____

Sleep/Other Notes

Date

Meals   Mood/ Physical Symptoms

Re-Introductions: _____

Digestion

BMs: _____

Sleep/ Other Notes

Date

Meals   Mood/Physical Symptoms

Re-Introductions:_____

Digestion

BMs: _____

Sleep/Other Notes

Date

Meals   Mood/ Physical Symptoms

Re-Introductions:_____

Digestion

BMs: _____

Sleep/ Other Notes

_____
_____

Date

Meals | Mood/Physical Symptoms

Re-Introductions:_____

Digestion

BMs: _____

Sleep/Other Notes

Date

Meals | Mood/ Physical Symptoms

Re-Introductions:_____

Digestion

BMs: _____

Sleep/ Other Notes

_____

_____

Date

Meals   Mood/ Physical Symptoms

❋

❋

❋

❋

Re-Introductions:_____

Digestion

BMs: _____

Sleep/ Other Notes

_____

_____

Date

Meals

Mood/ Physical Symptoms

❈

❈

❈

❈

Re-Introductions: _____

Digestion

BMs: _____

Sleep/ Other Notes

_____

_____

Date

Meals   Mood/ Physical Symptoms

Re-Introductions:_____

Digestion

BMs: _____

Sleep/ Other Notes

Date

Meals   ## Mood/Physical Symptoms

Re-Introductions:_____

Digestion

BMs: _____

Sleep/Other Notes

Date

Meals

Mood/ Physical Symptoms

Re-Introductions:_____

Digestion

BMs: _____

Sleep/ Other Notes

Date

Meals   ## Mood/Physical Symptoms

Re-Introductions: _____

Digestion

BMs: _____

Sleep/ Other Notes

Date

Meals   Mood/ Physical Symptoms

❖

❖

❖

❖

Re-Introductions: _____

Digestion

BMs: _____

Sleep/ Other Notes

_____

_____

Date

Meals

Mood/Physical Symptoms

Re-Introductions:_____

Digestion

BMs: _____

Sleep/Other Notes

Date

Meals   Mood/ Physical Symptoms

Re-Introductions:_____

Digestion

BMs: _____

Sleep/ Other Notes

Date

Meals

Mood/ Physical Symptoms

❄ _____

_____

❄ _____

_____

❄ _____

_____

❄ _____

Re-Introductions: _____

Digestion

BMs: _____

Sleep/ Other Notes

_____

_____

Date

Meals

Mood/ Physical Symptoms

❀

❀

❀

❀

Re-Introductions: _____

Digestion

BMs: _____

Sleep/ Other Notes

_____

_____

Date

Meals

Mood/ Physical Symptoms

Re-Introductions: _____

Digestion

BMs: _____

Sleep/ Other Notes

Date

Meals

Mood/ Physical Symptoms

Re-Introductions: _____

Digestion

BMs: _____

Sleep/ Other Notes

Date

Meals   Mood/ Physical Symptoms

Re-Introductions:_____

Digestion

BMs: _____

Sleep/ Other Notes

Date

Meals

Mood/ Physical Symptoms

Re-Introductions:_____

Digestion

BMs: _____

Sleep/ Other Notes

Date

Meals

Mood/Physical Symptoms

Re-Introductions: _____

Digestion

BMs: _____

Sleep/Other Notes

Date

Meals   Mood/ Physical Symptoms

_____
_____
_____
_____
_____
_____
_____
_____
_____
_____
_____
_____
_____
_____
_____

Re-Introductions:_____

Digestion

BMs: _____

Sleep/ Other Notes

_____
_____

Date

Meals   Mood/Physical Symptoms

❁

❁

❁

❁

Re-Introductions:_____

Digestion

BMs: _____

Sleep/Other Notes

Date

Meals   Mood/Physical Symptoms

❀

❀

❀

❀

Re-Introductions:_____

Digestion

BMs: _____

Sleep/Other Notes

Date

Meals	Mood/ Physical Symptoms

Re-Introductions:_____

Digestion

BMs: _____

Sleep/ Other Notes

Date

Meals   Mood/ Physical Symptoms

Re-Introductions:_____

Digestion

BMs: _____

Sleep/ Other Notes

Date

Meals

Mood/Physical Symptoms

Re-Introductions: _____

Digestion

BMs: _____

Sleep/Other Notes

Date

Meals   Mood/ Physical Symptoms

Re-Introductions:_____

Digestion

BMs: _____

Sleep/ Other Notes

_____

_____

Date

Meals

Mood/Physical Symptoms

Re-Introductions:_____

Digestion

BMs: _____

Sleep/Other Notes

Date

Meals   Mood/ Physical Symptoms

Re-Introductions: _____

Digestion

BMs: _____

Sleep/ Other Notes

Date

Meals   Mood/ Physical Symptoms

Re-Introductions: _____

Digestion

BMs: _____

Sleep/ Other Notes

Date

Meals

Mood/Physical Symptoms

Re-Introductions:_____

Digestion

BMs: _____

Sleep/Other Notes

Date

Meals

Mood/Physical Symptoms

❁

❁

❁

❁

Re-Introductions: _____

Digestion

BMs: _____

Sleep/Other Notes

Date

Meals   Mood/ Physical Symptoms

❁

❁

❁

❁

Re-Introductions:_____

Digestion

BMs: _____

Sleep/ Other Notes

Date

Meals   Mood/Physical Symptoms

Re-Introductions:_____

Digestion

BMs: _____

Sleep/Other Notes

_____

_____

Date

Meals   ## Mood/Physical Symptoms

Re-Introductions:_____

Digestion

BMs: _____

Sleep/Other Notes

Date

Meals   ## Mood/ Physical Symptoms

Re-Introductions: _____

Digestion

BMs: _____

Sleep/ Other Notes

Date

Meals   ## Mood/Physical Symptoms

Re-Introductions:_____

Digestion

BMs: _____

Sleep/Other Notes

Date

Meals

Mood/ Physical Symptoms

Re-Introductions:_____

Digestion

BMs: _____

Sleep/ Other Notes

Date

Meals

Mood/Physical Symptoms

Re-Introductions:_____

Digestion

BMs: _____

Sleep/Other Notes

_____

_____

Date

Meals   Mood/ Physical Symptoms

Re-Introductions: _____

Digestion

BMs: _____

Sleep/ Other Notes

Date

Meals   Mood/Physical Symptoms

Re-Introductions:_____

Digestion

BMs: _____

Sleep/Other Notes

_____

_____

Date

Meals

Mood/Physical Symptoms

Re-Introductions:_____

Digestion

BMs: _____

Sleep/Other Notes

Date

Meals   Mood/ Physical Symptoms

❀

❀

❀

❀

Re-Introductions:_____

Digestion

BMs: _____

Sleep/ Other Notes

_____

_____

Date

Meals   Mood/ Physical Symptoms

Re-Introductions:_____

Digestion

BMs: _____

Sleep/ Other Notes

Date

Meals   Mood/ Physical Symptoms

_____
_____
_____
_____
_____
_____
_____
_____
_____
_____
_____
_____
_____
_____
_____
_____

Re-Introductions: _____

Digestion

BMs: _____

Sleep/ Other Notes

_____
_____

Date

Meals   Mood/ Physical Symptoms

_____ ❁ _____
_____
_____
_____
_____ ❁ _____
_____
_____
_____
_____ ❁ _____
_____
_____
_____
_____ ❁ _____
_____
_____
_____

Re-Introductions:_____

Digestion

BMs: _____

Sleep/ Other Notes

_____
_____

Date

Meals   Mood/Physical Symptoms

Re-Introductions: _____

Digestion

BMs: _____

Sleep/Other Notes

_____

_____

Date

Meals   Mood/ Physical Symptoms

Re-Introductions:_____

Digestion

BMs: _____

Sleep/ Other Notes

Date

Meals   Mood/ Physical Symptoms

Re-Introductions: _____

Digestion

BMs: _____

Sleep/ Other Notes

Date

Meals

Mood/ Physical Symptoms

_____
_____
_____
_____
_____
_____
_____
_____
_____
_____
_____
_____
_____
_____
_____

Re-Introductions:_____

Digestion

BMs: _____

Sleep/ Other Notes

_____
_____

Date

Meals   ## Mood/ Physical Symptoms

_____
_____
_____
_____
_____
_____
_____
_____
_____
_____
_____
_____
_____
_____
_____
_____

Re-Introductions:_____

Digestion

BMs: _____

Sleep/ Other Notes

_____
_____

Date

Meals   Mood/ Physical Symptoms

_____
_____
_____
_____
_____
_____
_____
_____
_____
_____
_____
_____
_____

Re-Introductions:_____

Digestion

BMs: _____

Sleep/ Other Notes

_____
_____

Meals   *Mood/ Physical Symptoms*

Re-Introductions:_____

Digestion

BMs: _____

Sleep/ Other Notes

Date

Meals   Mood/ Physical Symptoms

_____
❁
_____
_____
_____
_____
❁
_____
_____
_____
_____
❁
_____
_____
_____
_____
❁
_____
_____
_____

Re-Introductions:_____

Digestion

BMs: _____

Sleep/ Other Notes

_____
_____

Date

Meals

Mood/ Physical Symptoms

❀

❀

❀

❀

Re-Introductions: _____

Digestion

BMs: _____

Sleep/ Other Notes

_____

_____

Date

Meals   Mood/ Physical Symptoms

_____
_____
_____
_____
_____
_____
_____
_____
_____
_____
_____
_____
_____
_____
_____
_____

Re-Introductions:_____

Digestion

BMs: _____

Sleep/ Other Notes

_____
_____

Date

Meals   Mood/ Physical Symptoms

Re-Introductions: _____

Digestion

BMs: _____

Sleep/ Other Notes

Date

Meals   ## Mood/ Physical Symptoms

_____
_____
_____
_____
_____
_____
_____
_____
_____
_____
_____
_____
_____
_____
_____
_____

Re-Introductions:_____

Digestion

BMs: _____

Sleep/ Other Notes

_____
_____

Meals

Mood/ Physical Symptoms

_____
❁
_____
_____
_____
_____
_____
❁
_____
_____
_____
_____
_____
❁
_____
_____
_____
_____
_____
❁
_____
_____
_____
_____

Re-Introductions:_____

Digestion

BMs: _____

Sleep/ Other Notes

_____

_____

Date

Meals

Mood/ Physical Symptoms

_____
_____
_____
_____
_____
_____
_____
_____
_____
_____
_____
_____
_____
_____
_____
_____

Re-Introductions:_____

Digestion

BMs: _____

Sleep/ Other Notes

_____
_____

Date

Meals   Mood/Physical Symptoms

_____
_____❁_____
_____
_____
_____
_____
_____❁_____
_____
_____
_____
_____
_____❁_____
_____
_____
_____
_____
_____❁_____
_____
_____
_____

Re-Introductions:_____

Digestion

BMs: _____

Sleep/Other Notes

_____
_____

Date

Meals   Mood/ Physical Symptoms

_____

_____

_____

_____

_____

_____

_____

_____

_____

_____

_____

_____

_____

_____

_____

Re-Introductions:_____

Digestion

BMs: _____

Sleep/ Other Notes

_____

_____

Meals   Mood/ Physical Symptoms

Re-Introductions:_____

Digestion

BMs: _____

Sleep/ Other Notes

Date

Meals   Mood/Physical Symptoms

_____
_____
_____
_____
_____
_____
_____
_____
_____
_____
_____
_____
_____
_____
_____
_____

Re-Introductions:_____

Digestion

BMs: _____

Sleep/Other Notes

_____
_____

Date

Meals   Mood/ Physical Symptoms

Re-Introductions: _____

Digestion

BMs: _____

Sleep/ Other Notes

Date

Meals

Mood/ Physical Symptoms

_____
_____
_____
_____
_____
_____
_____
_____
_____
_____
_____
_____
_____
_____
_____
_____

Re-Introductions:_____

Digestion

BMs: _____

Sleep/ Other Notes

_____
_____

Date

Meals   Mood/Physical Symptoms

Re-Introductions:_____

Digestion

BMs: _____

Sleep/Other Notes

Date

Meals   Mood/ Physical Symptoms

_____
_____
_____
_____
_____
_____
_____
_____
_____
_____
_____
_____
_____
_____
_____
_____

Re-Introductions:_____

Digestion

BMs: _____

Sleep/ Other Notes

_____
_____

Date

Meals   Mood/ Physical Symptoms

Re-Introductions:_____

Digestion

BMs: _____

Sleep/ Other Notes

Date

Meals   Mood/ Physical Symptoms

_____
_____
_____
_____
_____
_____
_____
_____
_____
_____
_____
_____
_____
_____
_____
_____

Re-Introductions:_____

Digestion

BMs: _____

Sleep/ Other Notes

_____
_____

Date

Meals

Mood/ Physical Symptoms

✿

✿

✿

✿

Re-Introductions: _____

Digestion

BMs: _____

Sleep/ Other Notes

_____

_____

Date

Meals

Mood/Physical Symptoms

Re-Introductions:_____

Digestion

BMs: _____

Sleep/Other Notes

Date

Meals   Mood/ Physical Symptoms

Re-Introductions:_____

Digestion

BMs: _____

Sleep/ Other Notes

_____

_____

Date

Meals   Mood/ Physical Symptoms

_____
_____
_____
_____
_____
_____
_____
_____
_____
_____
_____
_____
_____
_____
_____
_____

Re-Introductions:_____

Digestion

BMs: _____

Sleep/ Other Notes

_____
_____

Date

Meals

Mood/ Physical Symptoms

Re-Introductions:_____

Digestion

BMs: _____

Sleep/ Other Notes

Date

Meals

Mood/ Physical Symptoms

_____
_____
_____
_____
_____
_____
_____
_____
_____
_____
_____
_____
_____
_____
_____
_____

Re-Introductions:_____

Digestion

BMs: _____

Sleep/ Other Notes

_____
_____

Date

Meals   Mood/Physical Symptoms

Re-Introductions:_____

Digestion

BMs: _____

Sleep/Other Notes

Date

Meals

Mood/Physical Symptoms

Re-Introductions:_____

Digestion

BMs: _____

Sleep/Other Notes

Date

Meals   Mood/Physical Symptoms

_____
_____ ❁ _____
_____
_____
_____
_____
_____ ❁ _____
_____
_____
_____
_____ ❁ _____
_____
_____
_____
_____ ❁ _____
_____
_____
_____

Re-Introductions:_____

Digestion

BMs: _____

Sleep/Other Notes

_____
_____

Date

Meals   Mood/ Physical Symptoms

❁

❁

❁

❁

Re-Introductions: _____

Digestion

BMs: _____

Sleep/ Other Notes

_____

_____

Date

Meals   Mood/ Physical Symptoms

_____
✿ _____
_____
_____
_____
✿ _____
_____
_____
_____
✿ _____
_____
_____
_____
✿ _____
_____
_____

Re-Introductions:_____

Digestion

BMs: _____

Sleep/ Other Notes

_____
_____

Date

Meals

Mood/Physical Symptoms

_____
_____
_____
_____
_____
_____
_____
_____
_____
_____
_____
_____
_____
_____
_____
_____

Re-Introductions:_____

Digestion

BMs: _____

Sleep/Other Notes

_____
_____

Date

Meals

Mood/ Physical Symptoms

_____ ❀ _____
_____

_____
_____

_____ ❀ _____
_____

_____
_____

_____ ❀ _____
_____

_____
_____

_____ ❀ _____
_____

_____
_____

Re-Introductions:_____

Digestion

BMs: _____

Sleep/ Other Notes

_____
_____

Date

Meals   Mood/Physical Symptoms

Re-Introductions:_____

Digestion

BMs: _____

Sleep/ Other Notes

_____
_____

Date

Meals   Mood/ Physical Symptoms

_____

_____

_____

_____

_____

_____

_____

_____

_____

_____

_____

_____

_____

_____

_____

_____

Re-Introductions:_____

Digestion

BMs: _____

Sleep/ Other Notes

_____

_____

Date

Meals　　　　Mood/Physical Symptoms

_____
_____
_____
_____
_____
_____
_____
_____
_____
_____
_____
_____
_____
_____
_____
_____

Re-Introductions:_____

Digestion

BMs: _____

Sleep/Other Notes

_____
_____

Date

Meals

Mood/Physical Symptoms

Re-Introductions:_____

Digestion

BMs: _____

Sleep/Other Notes

Date

Meals

Mood/Physical Symptoms

Re-Introductions:_____

Digestion

BMs: _____

Sleep/Other Notes

Date

Meals   Mood/ Physical Symptoms

_____

_____

_____

_____

_____

_____

_____

_____

_____

_____

_____

_____

_____

_____

_____

_____

Re-Introductions:_____

Digestion

BMs: _____

Sleep/ Other Notes

_____

_____

Date

Meals   Mood/Physical Symptoms

_____
_____
_____
_____
_____
_____
_____
_____
_____
_____
_____
_____

Re-Introductions:_____

Digestion

BMs: _____

Sleep/Other Notes

_____
_____

Date

Meals   Mood/Physical Symptoms

❀

❀

❀

❀

Re-Introductions:_____

Digestion

BMs: _____

Sleep/Other Notes

_____

_____

Date

Meals   Mood/ Physical Symptoms

_____
_____
_____
_____
_____
_____
_____
_____
_____
_____
_____
_____
_____
_____
_____
_____

Re-Introductions:_____

Digestion

BMs: _____

Sleep/ Other Notes

_____
_____

Date

Meals   Mood/ Physical Symptoms

Re-Introductions:_____

Digestion

BMs: _____

Sleep/ Other Notes

Date

Meals   Mood/ Physical Symptoms

Re-Introductions:_____

Digestion

BMs: _____

Sleep/ Other Notes

Date

Meals   Mood/ Physical Symptoms

_____
❀ _____
_____
_____
_____
❀ _____
_____
_____
_____
❀ _____
_____
_____
_____
❀ _____
_____
_____
_____

Re-Introductions:_____

Digestion

BMs: _____

Sleep/ Other Notes

_____

_____

Date

Meals

Mood/ Physical Symptoms

Re-Introductions: _____

Digestion

BMs: _____

Sleep/ Other Notes

Date

Meals

Mood/ Physical Symptoms

❁

❁

❁

❁

Re-Introductions:_____

Digestion

BMs: _____

Sleep/ Other Notes

Date

Meals | Mood/Physical Symptoms

_____
_____
_____
_____
_____
_____
_____
_____
_____
_____
_____
_____
_____
_____
_____
_____

Re-Introductions:_____

Digestion

BMs: _____

Sleep/Other Notes

_____
_____

Date

Meals

Mood/ Physical Symptoms

Re-Introductions:_____

Digestion

BMs: _____

Sleep/ Other Notes

Date

Meals

Mood/Physical Symptoms

_____
_____
_____
_____
_____
_____
_____
_____
_____
_____
_____
_____
_____
_____
_____
_____

Re-Introductions:_____

Digestion

BMs: _____

Sleep/Other Notes

_____
_____

Date

Meals

Mood/ Physical Symptoms

Re-Introductions:_____

Digestion

BMs: _____

Sleep/ Other Notes

_____

_____

Meals   Mood/ Physical Symptoms

_____
_____
_____
_____
_____
_____
_____
_____
_____
_____
_____
_____
_____
_____
_____
_____

Re-Introductions:_____

Digestion

BMs: _____

Sleep/ Other Notes

_____
_____

Date

Meals

Mood/ Physical Symptoms

❁

❁

❁

❁

Re-Introductions:_____

Digestion

BMs: _____

Sleep/ Other Notes

_____

_____

Date

Meals | Mood/ Physical Symptoms

_____
_____
_____
_____
_____
_____
_____
_____
_____
_____
_____
_____
_____
_____
_____
_____

Re-Introductions:_____

Digestion

BMs: _____

Sleep/ Other Notes

_____
_____

Meals   Mood/Physical Symptoms

❁

❁

❁

❁

Re-Introductions: _____

Digestion

BMs: _____

Sleep/Other Notes

_____

_____

Date

Meals

Mood/Physical Symptoms

_____
_____
_____
_____
_____
_____
_____
_____
_____
_____
_____
_____
_____
_____
_____
_____
_____

Re-Introductions:_____

Digestion

BMs: _____

Sleep/Other Notes

_____
_____

Date

Meals   Mood/ Physical Symptoms

_____

⚘ _____

_____

_____

⚘ _____

_____

_____

⚘ _____

_____

_____

⚘ _____

_____

Re-Introductions:_____

Digestion

BMs: _____

Sleep/ Other Notes

_____

_____

Date

Meals

Mood/ Physical Symptoms

❀

❀

❀

❀

Re-Introductions:_____

Digestion

BMs: _____

Sleep/ Other Notes

Date

Meals

Mood/ Physical Symptoms

❀

❀

❀

❀

Re-Introductions: _____

Digestion

BMs: _____

Sleep/ Other Notes

Date

Meals   Mood/ Physical Symptoms

_____
_____
_____
_____
_____
_____
_____
_____
_____
_____
_____
_____
_____
_____
_____
_____
_____
_____

Re-Introductions:_____

Digestion

BMs: _____

Sleep/ Other Notes

_____
_____

Date

Meals   Mood/ Physical Symptoms

❁

❁

❁

❁

Re-Introductions: _____

Digestion

BMs: _____

Sleep/ Other Notes

_____

_____

Date

Meals

Mood/ Physical Symptoms

_____
_____
_____
_____
_____
_____
_____
_____
_____
_____
_____
_____
_____
_____
_____
_____

Re-Introductions:_____

Digestion

BMs: _____

Sleep/ Other Notes

_____
_____

Date

Meals   Mood/ Physical Symptoms

Re-Introductions:_____

Digestion

BMs: _____

Sleep/ Other Notes

Meals   Mood/ Physical Symptoms

_____
_____
_____
_____
_____
_____
_____
_____
_____
_____
_____
_____
_____
_____
_____
_____

Re-Introductions:_____

Digestion

BMs: _____

Sleep/ Other Notes

_____
_____

Date

Meals   Mood/ Physical Symptoms

Re-Introductions:_____

Digestion

BMs: _____

Sleep/ Other Notes

Date

Meals

Mood/Physical Symptoms

Re-Introductions:_____

Digestion

BMs: _____

Sleep/Other Notes

Date

Meals　　　　　Mood/ Physical Symptoms

❀

❀

❀

❀

Re-Introductions: _____

Digestion

BMs: _____

Sleep/ Other Notes

_____
_____

Date

Meals

Mood/ Physical Symptoms

Re-Introductions:_____

Digestion

BMs: _____

Sleep/ Other Notes

Date

Meals   Mood/ Physical Symptoms

Re-Introductions:_____

Digestion

BMs: _____

Sleep/ Other Notes

Date

Meals

Mood/ Physical Symptoms

_____

_____

_____

_____

_____

_____

_____

_____

_____

_____

_____

_____

_____

_____

_____

_____

Re-Introductions:_____

Digestion

BMs: _____

Sleep/ Other Notes

_____

_____

Date

Meals

Mood/Physical Symptoms

Re-Introductions: _____

Digestion

BMs: _____

Sleep/Other Notes

Date

Meals | Mood/ Physical Symptoms

_____
_____
_____
_____
_____
_____
_____
_____
_____
_____
_____
_____
_____
_____

Re-Introductions:_____

Digestion

BMs: _____

Sleep/ Other Notes

_____
_____

Date

Meals   Mood/ Physical Symptoms

❁

❁

❁

❁

Re-Introductions: _____

Digestion

BMs: _____

Sleep/ Other Notes

Date

Meals   Mood/ Physical Symptoms

_____
_____
_____
_____
_____
_____
_____
_____
_____
_____
_____
_____
_____
_____
_____
_____
_____

Re-Introductions:_____

Digestion

BMs: _____

Sleep/ Other Notes

_____
_____

Date

Meals   ## Mood/ Physical Symptoms

❁

❁

❁

❁

Re-Introductions:_____

Digestion

BMs: _____

Sleep/ Other Notes

Date

Meals   ## Mood/ Physical Symptoms

❀

❀

❀

❀

Re-Introductions: _____

Digestion

BMs: _____

Sleep/ Other Notes

_____

_____

Date

Meals   Mood/ Physical Symptoms

❈

❈

❈

❈

Re-Introductions:_____

Digestion

BMs: _____

Sleep/ Other Notes

_____

_____

Date

Meals

Mood/ Physical Symptoms

_____
_____
_____
_____
_____
_____
_____
_____
_____
_____
_____
_____
_____
_____
_____
_____

Re-Introductions:_____

Digestion

BMs: _____

Sleep/ Other Notes

_____
_____

Date

Meals   Mood/Physical Symptoms

Re-Introductions:

Digestion

BMs:

Sleep/Other Notes

Date

Meals

Mood/Physical Symptoms

Re-Introductions:_____

Digestion

BMs: _____

Sleep/Other Notes

_____
_____

Date

Meals   ## Mood/Physical Symptoms

Re-Introductions:

Digestion

BMs:

Sleep/Other Notes

Date

Meals   Mood/ Physical Symptoms

Re-Introductions: _____

Digestion

BMs: _____

Sleep/ Other Notes

Date

Meals

Mood/ Physical Symptoms

❀

❀

❀

❀

Re-Introductions: _____

Digestion

BMs: _____

Sleep/ Other Notes

_____

_____

Date

Meals   Mood/Physical Symptoms

Re-Introductions:_____

Digestion

BMs: _____

Sleep/Other Notes

Date

Meals   Mood/ Physical Symptoms

Re-Introductions:_____

Digestion

BMs: _____

Sleep/ Other Notes

Made in the USA
Lexington, KY
20 January 2019